Mériam SABBAH
Khadija MZOUGHI
Dalila GARGOURI

Evaluation of debriefing in endoscopic procedural simulation

Mériam SABBAH
Khadija MZOUGHI
Dalila GARGOURI

Evaluation of debriefing in endoscopic procedural simulation

ScienciaScripts

Imprint

Any brand names and product names mentioned in this book are subject to trademark, brand or patent protection and are trademarks or registered trademarks of their respective holders. The use of brand names, product names, common names, trade names, product descriptions etc. even without a particular marking in this work is in no way to be construed to mean that such names may be regarded as unrestricted in respect of trademark and brand protection legislation and could thus be used by anyone.

Cover image: www.ingimage.com

This book is a translation from the original published under ISBN 978-620-6-71808-6.

Publisher:
Sciencia Scripts
is a trademark of
Dodo Books Indian Ocean Ltd. and OmniScriptum S.R.L publishing group

120 High Road, East Finchley, London, N2 9ED, United Kingdom
Str. Armeneasca 28/1, office 1, Chisinau MD-2012, Republic of Moldova, Europe
Printed at: see last page
ISBN: 978-620-7-93558-1

INTRODUCTION

In gastroenterology, digestive endoscopy plays a central role in the training of future specialists. The quality of initial training will determine the quality of care delivered to the public. Practical training in digestive endoscopy, a procedure with considerable potential to cause harm [1], is an essential stage in the training of young gastroenterologists.At present, the learning of digestive endoscopy procedures and techniques is essentially carried out by a buddy system between an experienced endoscopist and his student. In order to overcome the disadvantages of this learning process (the principle of "never the first time on the patient" was not taken into consideration, major stress for the learners and danger for the patient), the current training of first-year gastroenterology residents begins with learning sessions on procedural simulators. There are typically four phases (briefing, simulator training, instant debriefing and assessment).Debriefing is a non-offensive, learner-centred conversation technique designed to help a professional or team improve performance through reflective practice [2]. It involves the active participation of learners, guided by a facilitator whose primary aim is to identify and address gaps in knowledge and skills [3].

These simulation sessions, which have recently been introduced into the curriculum of gastroenterology residents, have not yet been evaluated. particularly the debriefing phase, which is a crucial stage in clarifying and consolidating the learning acquired [4].

The Debriefing Assessment for Simulation in Healthcare (DASH) guide is a simple, easy and rapid multidimensional behavioural scale designed to assess and develop the debriefing skills of trainers and students using healthcare simulation. Hence the aim of our work, which was to evaluate debriefing in digestive endoscopy procedural simulation using the DASH tool (trainers and learners).

METHODS

1. POPULATION STUDIED :

1.1 Inclusion criteria :

We included first- and second-year gastroenterology residents who gave their consent to participate in the study and who completed the study questionnaire.

1.2 Non-inclusion criteria :

Third and fourth year residents were not included.

2. METHODS

2.1 Type, location and duration of study :

This was a cross-sectional study conducted at the Experimental Medicine Unit of the Tunis Faculty of Medicine over a period of four days (14-17 October 2019).

2.2 Description of equipment :

2.2.1 Simulators :

For our study, we used Koken® simulators for oesogastroduodenal endoscopy and colonoscopy (Figures 1 and 2).

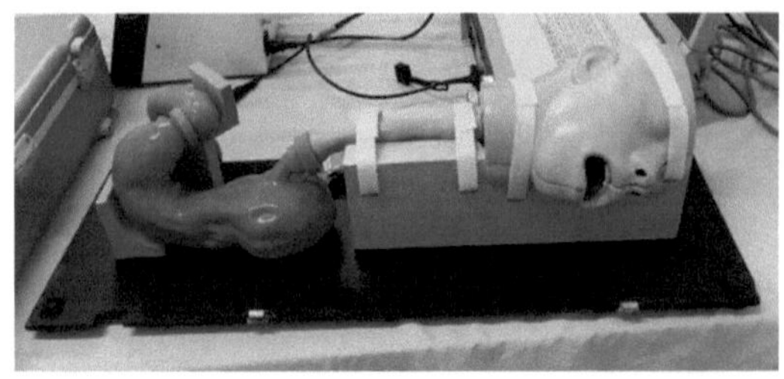

Figure 1: Koken oeso-gastroduodenal endoscopy simulator®

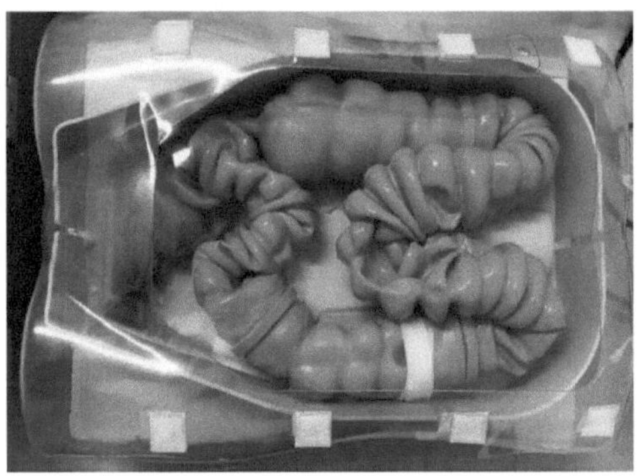

Figure 2: Koken colonoscopy simulator®

2.2.2 Endoscopy columns :

Digestive endoscopy columns and axial video endoscopes (fibroscopes and colonoscopes) specially dedicated to the simulation sessions were used. These were Karl Storz type endoscopes® (Figure 3).

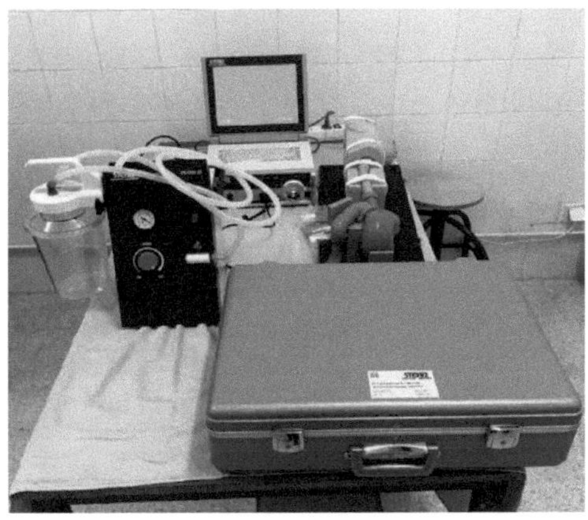

Figure 3: Case containing a Karl Storz type video endoscope® with portable aspirator and screen

2.3 Procedures :

The procedures performed during this training were diagnostic digestive endoscopy techniques, namely oesogastroduodenal endoscopy (EOGD) and colonoscopy.

2.4 Conduct of the study :

Our study was carried out as part of the Twin Training Course, which lasted four days. This is a cooperation between three countries: Tunisia, Germany and Egypt, with the aim of developing simulation-based learning in digestive endoscopy for gastroenterology residents in emerging countries. The training was given by university gastroenterologists with expertise in digestive endoscopy. There were five Tunisian trainers (one professor, two associate professors and two university hospital assistants), two Egyptians (one professor and one assistant) and five Germans (five professors). The simulation sessions took place in four phases for all participants: three formative (briefing, training on the simulator and debriefing) and one evaluative (Figure 4).

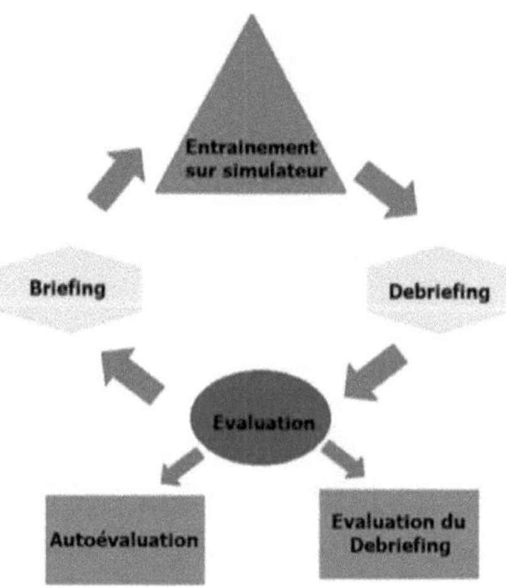

Figure 4: Loop sessions.

2.4.1 The formative phase :

2.4.1.1 Briefing:

The aim of this first phase was to introduce the participants to the objectives of the training course and how it would be run, to familiarise them with the procedural model and the tools to be used, and to describe the procedures to be carried out through demonstrations. The briefing session was carried out by all the trainers for the whole group. It lasted around 20 minutes and began with an introduction of the trainers and learners. The objectives of the training course, i.e. procedural simulation of upper and lower digestive endoscopy, were presented to the trainees. The procedure for the sessions (in groups of 3 or 4) was also explained, as well as the station-by-station rotation and the content of each station.

2.4.1.2 Training on the simulator :

Once the briefing was over, the participants were divided into groups of three or four for each station (EOGD or colonoscopy). This session lasted 1 to 2 hours. The trainer began by giving a demonstration, then each resident in turn performed a digestive endoscopy under the trainer's supervision and in front of their peers. This training was carried out according to Miller's skill pyramid (appendix 1) in four phases:

- First phase: the trainer performs the gesture without comment

- Second phase: the trainer performs the gesture and comments on it

- Third phase: the trainer performs the gesture and the learner comments on it.

- Fourth phase: the learner performs the gesture under the instructor's supervision

During this phase, the trainer constantly intervened to point out technical errors in the area of know-how and to ensure that the trainer was aware of them. showed the learner tips for optimising the performance of the exercise in progress (figure

5). Feedback and debriefing were instantaneous.

2.4.1.3 Debriefing:

During this phase, the trainer would review the session with the participants, summarising what they had learned and identifying the areas for improvement for each learner. This debriefing phase lasted 30 minutes. During this phase, the learners were first asked to express their feelings about the sessions, highlighting the strengths and weaknesses they perceived. Then, the trainers noted the different skills acquired by the learners and the improvements to be made in future sessions, as well as the objectives of the next simulation sessions. A final summary was produced.

2.4.2 The evaluation phase :

The evaluation consisted of two parts: an evaluation of the training by the residents and an evaluation of the debriefing.

2.4.2.1 Evaluation of the course by participants :

It was based on a self-questionnaire given out at the end of the session, comprising 21 questions (appendix 2):

- 20 questions about the course (assessed on a Lickert scale from 1 to 5),

- A question on their self-assessment of their progress before and after the course, using a skills scale graded from A to D (A very good, B satisfactory, C average, D poor),

2.4.2.2 Evaluation of the debriefing :

It was based on a self-questionnaire handed in at the end of the session. This self-questionnaire was based on the DASH evaluation grid in its two versions (trainer and learner).

In particular, the six elements of an effective debriefing following a simulation experience have been met. 7 The 6 sections of this scale refer to :

•Establish a climate favourable à learning (an engaging learning environment);

•Maintain a climate conducive to learning; - Conduct the debriefing in a structured manner;

•Encourage commitment in exchange (initiate interesting discussions) ;

•Identifying and exploring performance deficits ;

•Help learners acquire or maintain good practice. For each element, performance is graded on the basis of a Likert scale of seven levels of effectiveness: from 1, reflecting performance that is -extremely ineffective /detrimentall à the rating 7, corresponding à a performance judged-extremely effective/ exceptionall.

The two versions used (short versions) for trainers and learners are shown in

Appendices 3 and 4 respectively.

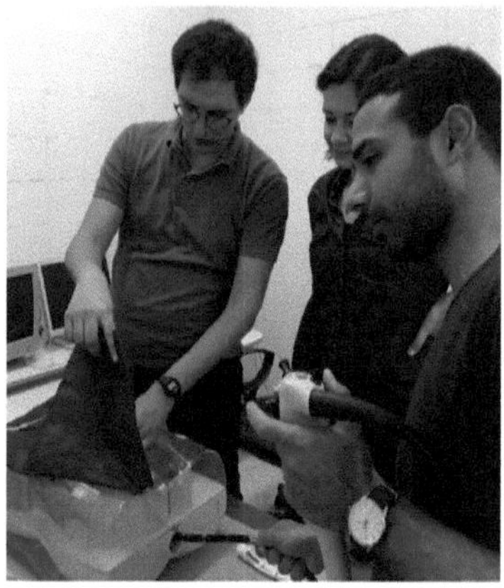

Figure 5: Gastroenterology residents simulating colonoscopy with a trainer

2.5 Statistical analysis :

The data were analysed using SPSS software® version 23.0.0.2.

2.5.1 Descriptive study :

For quantitative variables, we calculated the means and standard deviations, as well as the extreme values.

For qualitative variables, we calculated absolute and relative frequencies.

2.5.2 Analytical study :

The Wilcoxon test for paired samples was used to compare the scores for progress in acquiring digestive endoscopy skills. For all statistical tests, a p-value was considered statistically significant if less than 0.05.

2.6 Bibliographic research and reference management :

An automated bibliographic search was carried out on the Pubmed, Science Direct and Cochrane databases using the following key words: "Endoscopy", "Simulation", "Debriefing" and "Evaluation".We have consulted the articles in French and English. Bibliographic references were managed using Zotéro software® .

2.7 Ethical considerations :

Personal data was respected. In addition, the residents' consent was obtained for the use of their photographs in this simulation report. Informed consent in French was obtained from the residents before the study was carried out and after they had been provided with a letter of information about the aims of the study. The agreement of the Habib Thameur Hospital ethics committee was obtained for our study, which included residents (appendix 5).

2.8 Conflicts of interest and funding of the study :

We have no conflicts of interest to declare for this work. The simulators were purchased by the Tunis Faculty of Medicine. Endoscopes for dedicated use in training were loaned on a temporary basis. provided free of charge by Karl Stroz® . Small consumables were supplied free of charge by the trainers.

RESULTS

1. CHARACTERISTICS OF PARTICIPANTS :

Our study included fourteen gastroenterology residents.

1.1 Age and gender :

The average age of the participants was 26.5±1.6 years, with extremes ranging from 25 to 29 years. The gender ratio was 0.27 (3 men and 11 women).

1.2 Previous experience in digestive endoscopy :

Thirteen residents were in their first year and only one in his second year. All the residents had previous experience of upper GI endoscopy, while eight had previous experience of colonoscopy. These examinations were carried out independently or under the supervision of a senior. The average number of examinations previously carried out by residents is summarised in Table I.

Table I: Previous digestive endoscopies performed by residents

	Endoscopy upper digestive	Colonoscopy
On your own (median, extremes)	20 [0 - 50]	2,5 [0 - 20]
Under supervision (median, extremes)	17,5 [2 - 60]	3 [2 - 20]

2. STUDENT EVALUATION OF SIMULATION-BASED LEARNING :

2.1 Overall assessment of the course :

Overall, the residents were very satisfied with the training, with an overall average (out of five) for the various questions asked of 3.99±0.855 [1-5]. The responses to the self-questionnaire are summarised in Table II.

Table II: Overall assessment of training by residents

	Average	Standard deviation	Extremes
The objectives of training were clear and well-defined			[1 - 5]
	3,86	1,099	
The informationtransmitted was of good quality	3,71	0,825	[2 - 5]
The training content was in line with to your expectations			[2 - 5]
	3,43	0,756	
The stated objectives have been achieved	3,64	0,745	[2 - 5]
The activities were appropriate and useful	3,79	0,802	[2 - 5]
The trainers were available	4,36	0,929	[2 - 5]
The trainers created a climate conducive to learning	4,64	0,497	[4 - 5]
The general atmosphere was conducive to training	4,71	0,469	[4 - 5]
The duration of the course was sufficient	3,79	1,251	[1 - 5]
The size of the group was appropriate	4,00	1,240	[1 - 5]
The session made it easier for you to learn the basics about digestive endoscopy	4,21	0,802	[3 - 5]

2.2 **Overall assessment of participants' progress in acquiring competence in digestive endoscopy:**

A significant progression in the acquisition of digestive endoscopy skills after training was reported in the residents' self-assessment (p<0.0001). These results are summarised in Figure 6.

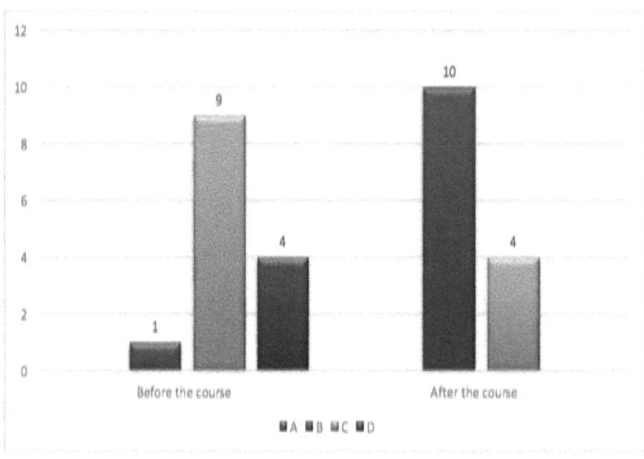

Figure6 :Overall in acquisition of in digestive endoscopy before and after training

*A very good level, B satisfactory level, C average level, D poor level.

Thirteen residents reported an increase in their skill level in their self-assessment. One resident felt that he had maintained the same level of competence before and after training (B). Individual progress is reported in table III.

Table III: Individual progress in acquiring competence in digestive endoscopy before and after training

		Competence after training		Total
		B	C	
Expertise before the course	B	1	0	1
	C	9	0	9
	D	1	3	4
Total		10	4	14

2.3 Debriefing evaluation :

The evaluation of the debriefing of the procedural simulation sessions was satisfactory overall, with respective averages of 4.67 to 6.6 and 4.22 and 6.22 for learners and trainers according to the scoring elements.The rating was slightly lower for learners on the element of identifying strengths and weaknesses (average of 4.67), and for trainers on the element of achieving and maintaining a good level of future performance (average of 4.22). The results of the DASH questionnaires for learners and trainers are shown in Tables IV and V respectively.

Table IV: Results of the DASH questionnaire for learners

	Average	Difference type	Extremes
The trainer has established a climate learning-friendly	6,26	0,431	[5 - 7]
The trainer maintained a climate conducive to learning	6,34	0,324	[5 - 7]
The trainer led the Structured debriefing	5,13	0,584	[4 - 6]
The trainer encouraged me to engage in discussion, which led me to analyse my performance	5,57	0,869	[5 - 7]
The trainer identified my strengths and areas for improvement, as well as the areas in need of improvement. reasons	4,67	0,267	[3 - 5]
The trainer helped me to think about how to improve or maintain a good level of performance	6,6	0,586	[5 - 7]

Table V: Results of the DASH questionnaire for trainers

	Average	Standard deviation	Extremes
Established a climate conducive to learning	6,16	0,224	[5 - 7]
Maintained a climate learning-friendly	6,22	0,124	[5 - 7]
Conducted the Debriefing of structured manner	5,47	0,547	[5 - 7]
Encouraged commitment to exchange	5,89	0,146	[5 - 7]
Identified and analysed performance gaps the reasons	4,22	0,259	[3 - 5]
Helped learners achieve or maintain a good level of language proficiency future performance	5,66	1,424	[4 - 7]

DISCUSSION

In gastroenterology, digestive endoscopy plays a central role in the training of future specialists, and the quality of initial training will determine the quality of care provided to the public.The introduction of learning digestive endoscopy through procedural simulation in the training of gastroenterology residents has been little evaluated, in particular the debriefing which has the particularity of being instantaneous in this setting. The aim of our work was to evaluate debriefing in digestive endoscopy procedural simulation using the DASH tool (trainers and learners).Our results showed that learning the basic techniques of digestive endoscopy using procedural model simulation improved the residents' technical performance in the short term, and the residents were satisfied with the learning method and their progress. It also showed that the debriefing was satisfactory from the point of view of learners and trainers, although there was room for improvement in terms of identifying strengths and weaknesses for learners and maintaining future performance levels for trainers. Our study is one of the first in Tunisia to assess the value of debriefing evaluation in simulation-based learning in digestive endoscopy. The main limitations of our study were :

- the small sample size,

- failure to use the long version of the DASH tool (more reliable)

- the lack of medium and long-term evaluation of the impact of the DASH questionnaire on the quality of debriefing during subsequent digestive endoscopy procedural simulation sessions.

1. THE SIMULATION PROCEDURAL IN GASTROENTEROLOGY :

Simulation is said to be procedural when it enables a precise technical gesture to be reproduced [5]. Complex procedural simulators can be used to reproduce more sophisticated interventional situations, such as digestive endoscopy or surgery [6]. They can be used by novice students, but also by experienced practitioners wishing to develop or diversify their skills. This learning method has a number of advantages, which increase with the realism of the simulator. It allows mastery of oculomotor control, self-assessment of performance and dexterity, and the acquisition of automatisms favoured by stress-free repetition of a technical gesture [7].

The tools available for training in digestive endoscopy are organic, inorganic and hybrid simulation. As far as organic simulation is concerned, most digestive endoscopy training is carried out on animal models (explanted live organs, mainly the EASIE pig stomach model) or on live animals [8,9]. These models have been used in Tunisia as part of one-off training courses with foreign experts or as part of digestive endoscopy workshops. In fact, their transport and Their delicate use, in addition to their short lifespans, make them difficult models to transpose into the daily training of residents. Non-organic simulation includes synthetic models, such as dedicated mannequins, and electronic models, which present a natural (virtual reality) interface combining an endoscope with an electronic interface reproducing digestive anatomy, physiology and pathology [10]. These are the models mainly used in the current training of gastroenterology residents.Finally, hybrid simulation combines different simulation techniques: for example, a standardised patient is used to assess communication, then a procedural simulator is used to simulate a technical procedure. This method is well-suited to learning both know-how and interpersonal skills, as it allows us to assess communication with the patient (before and after the procedure) and teamwork.

During our training, we used the synthetic model because of its advantages: lower cost, ease of use, good technicality with the possibility of repeating simple and fairly complex gestures, and a good lifespan [18]. The limitation of this simulator is that it is not suitable for assessing interpersonal skills.

2. THE BENEFITS OF SIMULATION DEBRIEFING :

2.1 Definition of debriefing and the different stages:

Debriefing is a crucial stage in clarifying and consolidating the learning acquired from simulation experiences in the healthcare field [4].

It is a non-offensive, learner-centred conversation technique designed to help a professional or team improve performance through reflective practice [11]. It involves the active participation of learners, guided by a facilitator or instructor whose aim is to identify and address gaps in knowledge and skills [3].

A debriefing must be structured, factual and objective, specific and precise in order to guarantee objectivity [12]. Structured debriefing usually involves three phases (descriptive, analysis and summary phases), taking into account the pedagogical objectives 12 and maintaining a favourable learning climate (climate of trust, psychological safety) [13].

During the descriptive phase, the trainer gathers "on-the-spot" reactions (experiences, frustrations, difficulties, negative emotions) [14] and clarifies the learners' expectations. The trainer then encourages and guides the description (how the session went, coordination of actions, communication, how the team functioned, activities that were thought of but not carried out). They encourage all the learners to participate and stimulate discussion (active listening).

During the analysis phase, the trainer methodically examines what happened and why, encouraging learners to self-correct. He clarifies the learning objectives. He validates what has been learnt and corrects errors (remediable behaviours), suggests alternative "solutions" and checks that the learners have understood correctly [15]. During the wrap-up phase, the trainer reviews the key points of the session. He summarises the positive points of the session, the points to be worked on and the improvements identified during the scenario (Take Home Messages) [15].

2.2 Evaluation tools for simulation debriefing :

Conducting a debriefing of a simulation session requires a particular skill which can be improved by feedback [16]. This feedback therefore requires adequate training for the trainers, followed by periodic evaluation for training purposes. This evaluation can be carried out by learners, peers or by self-evaluation. Learners assess the welcome they receive, the teaching resources and methods used, and the extent to which learning objectives have been achieved. Debriefing evaluation is based on specific evaluation grids, direct observation of practices or videos of simulation and debriefing sessions [17].

Various evaluation scales have been developed with a view to improving teaching practices. They are designed to help assess and develop the skills needed to conduct a debriefing. The main tools available for evaluating debriefing are shown in Table VI.

Table VI: Main evaluation tools for simulation debriefing

Tool	DASH	OSAD*	DES	PADI***
ement s	Establishes a climate conducive to learning Maintains a climate conducive to learning Structured debriefing Engages learners in discussion Identifies and explores performance gaps Helps learners achieve and maintain good performance	Approach (caring) Learning environment Learner engagement Learner reaction Reflection Analysis of causes underlying actions Diagnosis of performance and shortcomings Application (transfer to future practice)	Analysis of reasoning and feelings Learning and creating links (connections) Skills of the facilitator in leading the debriefing Adequate supervision by the facilitator	Organisation of the debriefing Verbal and non-verbal communication Setting the scene and the ground rules for debriefing Talking about emotions Summarising the experience Structure and reflection-in-action (facilitating the learner's self-reflection) Facilitating connections from experience to practice clinic
Summarise and provide key messages.				
Quotation	7-point Lickert scale points	5-point Lickert scale points	5-point Lickert scale points	4-point Lickert scale points

*OSAD: Objective Structure Assessment of Debriefing

**DES: Debriefing experience scale

***PADI: Peer Assessment Debriefing Instrument

Other methods also exist, such as video-debriefing. This involves small group sessions with simulation educators in which video segments of individual debriefing performances can be commented on, reflected upon and discussed in order to give constructive feedback [18].

2.3 Interest of the DASH tool in Debriefing evaluation

This scale was designed by the team at the Center for Medical Simulation in Boston on the basis of a review of the literature and recommendations for good debriefing practice from a group of 136 international experts[20].

It is the most widely used and best validated scale for assessing the quality of debriefings, due to its ease and simplicity of use. Its reliability, internal consistency, high inter-rater reproducibility and validity have been well demonstrated by several studies [11,21].

Although, from an evaluation point of view, this scale contains subjective elements, it remains a useful guide to ensure that facilitators respect the principles of debriefing [22]. The DASH is a behavioural assessment scale with qualitative descriptors which explores 6 essential elements of debriefing: establishing a climate conducive to learning, maintaining a climate conducive to learning, conducting the debriefing in a structured way, encouraging engagement in the exchange, identifying gaps in performance and analysing the reasons for them, helping learners to achieve or maintain a good level of future performance. We chose to use the short version of the DASH scale, as the long version contains a total of 23 behaviours which are rated on a 7-point Likert scale (1 = Extremely ineffective / detrimental to 7 = Extremely effective / exceptional), which we felt was longer and more difficult for participants to complete. The DASH exists in 3 versions: trainer, learner and trainer assessor.

The latter was not used in our study. The use of the dual trainer and learner version is a strong point of our work, enabling trainers to become aware of and acclimatise to the outside view of their debriefing (DASH learners), and a self-assessment (DASH trainer). This makes it possible to seek solutions to the difficulties encountered by setting up 'debriefing of the debriefing' sessions based on the trainers' self-confrontation and reflection on their performance.A study published in 2016 [23], assessing the value of the DASH in evaluating the debriefing of newborn resuscitation simulation sessions in the delivery room, included 156 participants. This The study concluded that learners evaluated the debriefings by high-level DASHs, validating the pedagogical framework of the programme. Conversely, the DASH trainers were heterogeneous and weaker. According to this work, conducting debriefings remained a complex exercise. The use of the DASH is part of a reflective approach by trainers to their own practice [24].

2.4 Particularities of procedural simulation and Tunisian data

Debriefing in procedural simulation has the particularity of being instantaneous during the different stages of procedural simulation, and trainers are led to carry out a debriefing after each station or each performance of a technical gesture in order to anchor the acquisition of performance in the learners. This makes it more difficult to evaluate [25,26].

On reviewing the Tunisian literature, we did not find any Tunisian studies on the subject, particularly on debriefing and its evaluation in procedural simulation. However, a Tunisian study published in February 2018 [27] had already proposed, in an evaluation grid for simulation trainers, to include the DASH in the evaluation of the debriefing, stressing the constructive and formative nature of the latter. The part of the debriefing evaluation proposed by this Tunisian evaluation grid is shown in appendix 6. This grid included the evaluation of the three phases of the debriefing, i.e. the descriptive phase, the analysis phase and the summary phase, with items rated (done/not done). This study concluded that simulation trainers need to acquire the skills required to manage simulation sessions and, more particularly, debriefing, which can pose certain difficulties because it requires a certain mastery of interpersonal skills. This requires specific initial training, of course, but also regular assessment of practices. This evaluation had a beneficial effect on their teaching practices, leading to improvements.

3.OUTLOOK :

At the end of our study, we recommended that the use of the DASH tool during procedural simulation sessions for learning endoscopy (both diagnostic and therapeutic) be generalised for all gastroenterology residents, incorporating different levels of complexity depending on the resident's level (diagnostic endoscopy for 1ère and 2ème year residents and therapeutic endoscopy for 3ème and 4ème year residents). The first step would be to train the trainers to carry out a structured debriefing at the end of each simulation session. This would make it possible to define the improvement actions to be undertaken by the trainers. We therefore propose to use this DASH questionnaire (trainers and learners, and subsequently trainers' assessors) at the end of each simulation session and to reassess the improvement in the quality of the debriefing over the sessions, particularly in terms of assessing the points to be improved and maintaining performance.

Simulation is currently an active learning method which is playing an increasingly important role in medical training, particularly in the acquisition of basic techniques of digestive endoscopy. Hence the recent development of procedural simulation, which makes it possible to learn endoscopy while respecting ethical principles, in particular the famous "never the first time on the patient" principle. The development of an experimental sciences unit at the Tunis Faculty of Medicine, which includes several models of procedural simulation in digestive endoscopy, has made it possible to introduce procedural simulation into the curriculum of first- and second-year gastroenterology residents. Among the stages of healthcare simulation, debriefing is recognised as a fundamental part of the learning process. What makes it special in procedural simulation is that it is instantaneous. The Debriefing Assessment for Simulation in Healthcare (DASH) guide, in its trainers and students version, is a tool designed to assess and develop the debriefing skills of trainers using healthcare simulation.Its short version is easy to use, enabling real-time evaluation of debriefing in procedural simulation.This is the background to our work, the aim of which was to evaluate debriefing in procedural simulation in digestive endoscopy using the DASH tool (trainer and student). To do this, we carried out a cross-sectional study including fourteen gastroenterology residents who took part in a four-day training course in digestive endoscopy at the experimental medicine unit of the Faculty of Medicine in Tunis from 14 to 17 October. 2019. Residents in their 3ème or 4ème year were not included in the study. The procedural simulation models used were of the synthetic type (Koken®) and the endoscopy columns of the type (Karl Storz®). The procedures evaluated were upper digestive endoscopy and colonoscopy. The simulation sessions took place in four phases for all participants: three formative (briefing, training on the simulator with immediate feedback and debriefing) and one evaluative.All sessions were supervised by trainers experienced in digestive endoscopy and familiar with the procedures to be carried out. The evaluation of the session included a self-assessment sheet and a debriefing evaluation. The self-assessment form consisted of 20 questions on the course of the training (assessed on a Lickert scale from 1 to 5), one question on the self-assessment of their progress before and after the training on a competence scale rated from A to D (A very good level, B satisfactory level, C average level, D poor level). The evaluation of the debriefing of the sessions was carried out using the DASH tool for the trainers and for the students in its short version (with six items respectively).Informed consent was obtained from the residents after they had been provided with a letter of information about the aims of the study. The agreement of the Habib Thameur Hospital ethics committee was obtained for the study. Our study included fourteen residents with a mean age of 26.5±1.6 years and a gender ratio of 0.27. Thirteen residents were in and one in the second year. All the residents h a d previous experience of upper GI endoscopy, while eight had previous experience of colonoscopy. Overall, the residents were very satisfied with the training, with an overall average (out of five) for the various questions asked of 3.99±0.855. A significant progression in the acquisition of digestive endoscopy skills after training was reported in the residents' self-assessment (p<0.0001). One resident felt that he had maintained the same level of competence before and after training. The evaluation of the debriefing of the procedural simulation sessions was satisfactory overall, with respective averages of 4.67 to 6.6 and 4.22 and 6.22 for learners and trainers according to the scoring elements. The rating was slightly lower for learners on the element of identifying strengths and weaknesses (average of 4.67), and for trainers on the element of achieving and maintaining a good level of future performance (average of 4.22). Our results are in line with those in the literature, which have shown that procedural simulation not only improves learners' performance in endoscopy in a safe context. In addition, the learners were satisfied with this learning method. In addition, they confirm the value of the DASH tool in evaluating the debriefing of simulation sessions, even if improvements are needed to emphasise the analysis of the learners' strengths and areas for improvement, and in maintaining a good level of future performance for the trainers. The main limitations of our study were :

- the small sample size,

- failure to use the long version of the DASH tool (more reliable)

- the lack of medium and long-term evaluation of the impact of the DASH

questionnaire on the quality of debriefing during subsequent digestive

endoscopy procedural simulation sessions.

Finally, at the end of our pilot study, learning basic digestive endoscopy

techniques using procedural model simulation improved the residents' technical

performance in the short term, and they were satisfied with their progress. The

evaluation of the debriefing showed satisfactory results from the point of view of

both trainers and learners. This evaluation is an essential step in the simulation

learning process and it would be wise to generalise it during procedural

simulation sessions in digestive endoscopy in order to improve the quality of the

sessions, to identify the strong and weak points of the learners, and to optimise

the performance of the trainers.

REFERENCES

1. Alinier G. A typology of educationally focused medical simulation tools. Med Teach;29(8):e243-50.

2. Michaela Kolbe, Bastian Grande, Donat R.Spahn. Briefing and debriefing during . simulation-based training and beyond: content, structure, attitude and setting. 2015 Best Practice and Research Clinical Anesthesiology 29, 87-96

3. Cheng A., Grant V., Huffman J., Burgess G., Szyld D., Robinson T., Eppich W.Coaching the debriefer: peer coaching to improve debriefing quality in simulation programs 2017. Simulation in Healthcare : The Journal of the Society for Simjulation in Healthcare Volume 12, Issue 5, 319-325

4. Dufrene, C., & Young, A. (2014). Successful debriefing - Best methods to achieve positive learning outcomes: A literature review. Nurse Education Today, 34(3), 372-376.

5. Issenberg SB, McGaghie WC, Hart IR, Mayer JW, Felner JM, Petrusa ER et al. Simulation technology for health care professional skills training and assessment. JAMA.1999;282(9):861-6.

6. Miller KK, Riley W, Davis S, Hansen HE. In Situ Simulation A Method of Experiential Learning to Promote Safety and Team Behavior. J Perinat Neonat Nurs. 2008;22(2):105-13.

7. Cook DA, Hatala R, Brydges R, Zendejas B, Szostek JH, Wang AT et al.Technology-enhanced simulation for health professions education: a

systematic review and meta-analysis. JAMA. 2011;306(9):978-88

8. Parra-Blanco A, González N, González R, Ortiz-Fernández-SordoJ, Ordieres C. Animal models for endoscopic training: do we really need them? Endoscopy. 2013;45(6):478-84.

9. Jones MW, Deere MJ, Harris JR, Chen AJ, Henning WH. Fabrication of An Inexpensive but Effective Colonoscopic Simulator. JSLS. 2017;21(2):e2017.00002.

10. Dray X, Camus M, Marteau P. Teaching endoscopy on an electronic simulator. Acta Endosc. 2013 ;43(5-6):283-92.

11. Brett-Fleegler M, Rudolph J, Eppich W, et al. Debriefing assessment for simulation in healthcare. Development and psychometric properties. Simul Healthc 2012;7:288-94.

12. Antonia Blaniea Morgan. Debriefing values in high - fidelity simulation. 2017 Anesthesia Critical Care and Pain Medicine, volume 36, issue 4, 201-202

13. Rudolph JW, Raemer DB, Simon R. Establishing a safe container for learning in simulation: the role of the presimulation brief- ing. Sim Healthc 2014;9:339-49.

14. Tannenbaum SI, Cerasoli CP. Do team and individual debriefs enhance performance? A meta-analysis. Hum Factors 2013 February 1;55:231e45.

15. Salas, E., Klein, M. S., King, H., Salisbury, M., Augenstein, J. S., Birnbach, D. J., & Upshaw, C. (2008). Debriefing medical teams: 12 evidence-based best practices and tips. The Joint Commission Journal on Quality and Patient Safety,

34(9), 518-527.

16. Hall K., Tori K. Best Practice Recommendations for Debriefing in Simulation-Based Education for Australian Udergraduate Nursing Students: An Integrative Review. 2016 Clinical Simulation in Nursing 1-12

17. Kam AJ, Gonsalves CL, Nordlund SV, Hale SJ, Twiss J, Cupido C et al. Implementation and facilitation of post-resuscitation debriefing: a comparative crossover study of two post-resuscitation debriefing frameworks. BMC Emerg Med. 2022 Sep;22(1):152

18. Cheng A, Grant V, Dieckmann P, et al. Faculty development for simulation programs: five issues for the future of debriefing training. Sim Healthc 2015;10:217-22.

19. Annette R. Waznonis Methods and Evaluation for Simulation Debriefing in Nursing Education. 2014. J.Nurs Educ 53(8) :459-465

20. Simon R, Raemer DB, Rudolph JW. Debriefing Assessment for Simulation in Healthcare. Boston, MA: Center for Medical Simulation; 2010- 2011 Available on the Harvard website https://harvardmedsim.org/dash-fr.ph and -https://harvardmedsim.org/_media/DASH_Manuel_utilisation_2010_VF_12-07.pdf. http://www.harvardmedsim.org/debriefing-assesment-simulation-healthcare.php

21. Dreifuerst KT. Using debriefing for meaningful learning to foster development of clinical reasoning in simulation. J Nurs Educ. 2012 Jun; 51(6): 326-33.

22. Oriot D., Alinier G. La simulation en santé. Le débriefing clé en mains. 2019 Elsevier Masson

23. Durand C, Secheresse T, Leconte M. The use of the Debriefing Assessment for Simulation in Healthcare (DASH) in a simulation-based team learning program for newborn resuscitation in the delivery room. Arch Pediatr. 2017 Dec;24(12):1197-1204.

24. Thompson R, Sullivan S, Campbell K, Osman I, Statz B, Jung HS. Does a Written Tool to Guide Structured Debriefing Improve Discourse? Implications for Interprofessional Team Simulation. J Surg Educ. 2018 Nov;75(6):e240-5.

25. Hunter LA. Debriefing and Feedback in the Current Healthcare Environment. J Perinat Neonatal Nurs. 2016 Jul- Sep;30(3):174-8.

26. Rudolph JW, Simon R, Raemer DB, Eppich WJ. Debriefing as formative assessment: closing performance gaps in medical education. Acad Emerg Med. 2008 Nov;15(11):1010-6.

27. I. Ben Amor, Y.Hentati, J. Gargouri. Evaluation grids for health simulation trainers 2018. J.I.M.Sfax N°28 ;1-9

APPENDICES

35

Appendix 1: MILLER skills pyramid

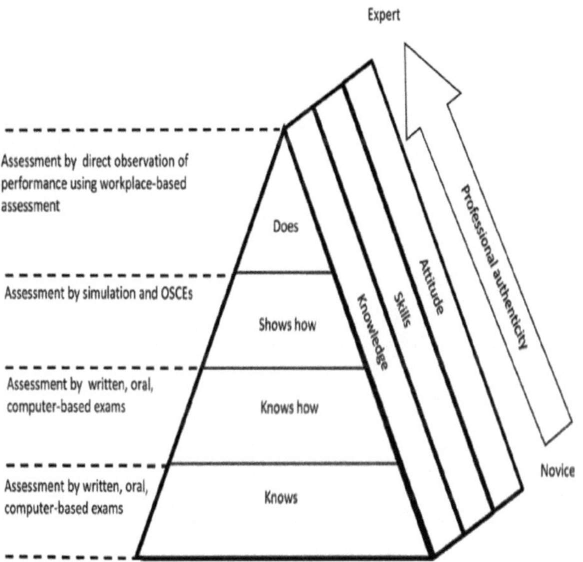

Appendix 2: Data collection template

Code

Seminar evaluation form: Twin Training Course 14 to 17 October 2019

Dear residents

You have just taken part in procedural simulation training in digestive

endoscopy.

Please complete the evaluation form so that we can improve and add to the list

of training courses on offer.

NB: The evaluation is anonymous Thank you for your cooperation

AgeSex MFResident in : 1ère year 2ème year

Your course: internships completed

Semester 1

Semester 2

Semester 3

Semester 4

Have you ever done :

- Upper digestive endoscopy yes no

If yes independently(number=)under supervision (number =)

- Colonoscopies yes no

If yes independently (number=)under supervision (number =)

I/ Overall assessment :

1. The training objectives were clear and well defined **Strongly** disagree1 2 3

45Strongly agree

2. The information provided was of good quality

Strongly disagree1 2 3 4 5 Strongly agree

3. The content of the training was in line with my expectations **Strongly**

disagree1 2 3 4 5 Totally agree

4. The objectives announced have been achieved

Strongly disagree1 2 3 4 5 Strongly agree

5. The activities were appropriate and useful

Strongly disagree1 2 3 4 5 Strongly agree

6. The trainers were available

Strongly disagree1 2 3 4 5 Strongly agree

7. The trainers have established a climate conducive to learning

Strongly disagree 1 2 3 4 5 Strongly agree

8. The general atmosphere was conducive to training

Strongly disagree 1 2 3 4 5 Strongly agree

9. The duration of the training was sufficient

Strongly disagree 1 2 3 4 5 Strongly agree

10. The size of the group was adequate

Strongly disagree 1 2 3 4 5 Strongly agree

11. Acquire the fundamentals of digestive endoscopy more easily

Strongly disagree 1 2 3 4 5 Strongly agree

12. Assessment of your progress in acquiring competence in digestive endoscopy (ascending from D to A)

Skill level prior to training: D	C	B	A
Skill level after training: D	C	B	A

Appendix 3: DASH questionnaire for trainers (short version)

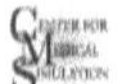

L'élément 1 évalue l'introduction (le briefing) de la séquence de simulation. Les éléments 2 à 6 évaluent le débriefing.

Echelle de notation :

Notation	1	2	3	4	5	6	7
Description	Extrêmement inefficace / préjudidable	Toujours inefficace / mauvais	Généralement inefficace / médiocre	Assez efficace / moyen	Généralement efficace / bon	Toujours efficace / très bon	Extrêmement efficace / exceptionnel

L'**élément 1 évalue l'introduction (le briefing) de la séquence de simulation.** *Passez cet élément si vous n'avez pas fait d'introduction.*

Elément 1	Note élément 1
J'ai établi un climat favorable à l'apprentissage	

- Je me suis présenté(e), ai décrit l'environnement de la simulation, expliqué ce qui était attendu au cours de la séance, annoncé les objectifs pédagogiques et clarifié les questions de confidentialité
- J'ai expliqué les points forts et les points faibles de la simulation et ce que les apprenants pouvaient faire pour tirer le meilleur parti des expériences de simulation clinique
- J'ai précisé les détails logistiques, comme l'emplacement des toilettes, les possibilités de restauration, et le déroulement de la journée, …
- J'ai encouragé les apprenants à exprimer leurs réflexions et leurs questions au sujet de la simulation et du débriefing à venir et les ai rassurés sur le fait qu'ils ne seraient ni mortifiés ni humiliés dans cet exercice.

Les éléments 2 à 6 évaluent le débriefing.

Elément 2	Note élément 2
J'ai maintenu un climat favorable à l'apprentissage	

- J'ai clarifié les objectifs du débriefing, ce qui était attendu de la part des apprenants et précisé mon rôle (en tant que formateur) dans le débriefing
- J'ai reconnu les inquiétudes des apprenants au sujet du réalisme des situations simulées et je les ai aidés à apprendre, malgré les limites de la simulation
- J'ai fait preuve de respect envers les apprenants
- J'ai assuré que l'apprentissage était l'objectif principal de la séance et non pas la stigmatisation des apprenants ayant commis des erreurs
- J'ai encouragé les apprenants à exprimer leurs réflexions et leurs émotions sans crainte d'être mortifiés ou humiliés

<table>
<tr><td>Elément 3</td><td align="right">Note élément 3</td></tr>
<tr><td colspan="2">J'ai conduit le débriefing de manière structurée</td></tr>
</table>

- J'ai guidé les échanges de façon à ce qu' ils progressent de façon logique plutôt que de passer d'un point à un autre sans cohérence
- Vers le début du débriefing, j'ai encouragé les apprenants à partager leur ressenti et j'ai pris en compte leurs remarques
- Au cours de la séance, j'ai aidé les apprenants à analyser leurs actions et les processus cognitifs qu'ils ont mis en œuvre
- A la fin du débriefing, j'ai réalisé une synthèse au cours de laquelle j'ai aidé les apprenants à faire des liens entre les différentes notions explorées et j'ai relié la séance de simulation aux façons dont les apprenants pourraient améliorer leur pratique clinique future

<table>
<tr><td>Elément 4</td><td align="right">Note élément 4</td></tr>
<tr><td colspan="2">J'ai suscité l'engagement dans l'échange, ce qui les a amenés à analyser leur performance</td></tr>
</table>

- J'ai utilisé des exemples concrets (pas seulement des commentaires abstraits ou généralistes) pour amener les apprenants à réfléchir sur leur performance
- Mon propos était clair ; je n'ai pas obligé les apprenants à imaginer mes pensées
- J'ai écouté et amené les personnes à se sentir entendues, en étant attentif à chacune, en reformulant leur propos, et en utilisant un langage non verbal adapté (par exemple, en regardant dans les yeux ou par des hochements de tête)
- J'ai utilisé la vidéo ou d'autres enregistrements à bon escient comme support pour les échanges et l'apprentissage
- Si l'un des apprenants s'est senti contrarié ou émotionnellement troublé lors du débriefing, j'ai été respectueux et constructif en l'aidant à gérer ses émotions

<table>
<tr><td>Elément 5</td><td align="right">Note élément 5</td></tr>
<tr><td colspan="2">J'ai identifié les points forts et les points à améliorer et leurs raisons</td></tr>
</table>

- J'ai fourni des feedbacks constructifs aux apprenants à propos de leur performance individuelle ou collective en m'appuyant sur des faits concrets et sur mon point de vue sincère
- J'ai aidé les apprenants à explorer ce qu'ils pensaient ou tentaient de mettre en œuvre à des moments clés

<table>
<tr><td>Elément 6</td><td align="right">Note élément 6</td></tr>
<tr><td colspan="2">Je les ai aidés à envisager comment améliorer ou maintenir un bon niveau de performance</td></tr>
</table>

- J'ai aidé les apprenants à apprendre comment améliorer leurs points faibles ou comment maintenir une bonne performance
- J'ai utilisé mon expertise dans le domaine traité pour aider les apprenants à voir comment améliorer leur performance dans une situation future
- Je me suis assuré(e) que les points importants avaient été abordés

Appendix 4: DASH questionnaire for learners (long version)

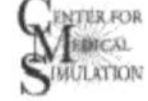

Consignes : Veuillez résumer votre impression de l'introduction et du débriefing de la séance de simulation. Utilisez l'échelle de notation suivante pour évaluer les 6 « éléments ». Chaque élément comprend les « comportements » signalés. Si l'un des critères ne peut être évalué (par exemple, comment le formateur a géré les personnes contrariées ou émotionnellement troublées, si personne ne l'a été), ne le laissez pas influencer votre évaluation. Le formateur peut avoir été à la fois performant et moins performant au sein d'un même élément. Faites de votre mieux pour **évaluer d'un point de vue *global* chaque élément**, guidé par votre observation des comportements qui le composent.

Echelle de notation :

Notation	1	2	3	4	5	6	7
Description	Extrêmement inefficace / préjudiciable	Toujours inefficace / mauvais	Généralement inefficace / médiocre	Assez efficace / moyen	Généralement efficace / bon	Toujours efficace / très bon	Extrêmement efficace / exceptionnel

L'élément 1 évalue l'introduction (le briefing) de la séquence de simulation. *(Passez cet élément si vous n'avez pas participé à l'introduction). S'il n'y a pas eu d'introduction et que celle-ci vous aurait paru indispensable, vous devez noter l'élément.*

Elément 1 Le formateur a établi un climat favorable à l'apprentissage	Note globale élément 1

- Le formateur s'est présenté, a décrit l'environnement de la simulation, expliqué ce qui était attendu au cours de la séance, et annoncé les objectifs pédagogiques
- Le formateur a expliqué les points forts et les points faibles de la simulation et m'a indiqué ce que je pouvais faire pour tirer le meilleur parti d'une expérience de simulation clinique
- Le formateur a précisé les détails logistiques, comme l'emplacement des toilettes, les possibilités de restauration, le déroulement de la journée, …
- Le formateur m'a encouragé(e) à exprimer mes réflexions et mes questions au sujet de la simulation et du débriefing à venir et m'a rassuré(e) sur le fait que je ne serais ni mortifié(e) ni humilié(e) dans cet exercice

Les éléments 2 à 6 évaluent le débriefing.

Elément 2 Le formateur a maintenu un climat favorable à l'apprentissage	Note globale élément 2

- Le formateur a clarifié les objectifs du débriefing, ce qu'il attendait de moi et précisé son rôle (en tant que formateur) dans le débriefing
- Le formateur a reconnu des inquiétudes au sujet du réalisme des situations simulées et m'a aidé(e) à apprendre, malgré les limites de la simulation
- J'ai constaté que le formateur a fait preuve de respect vis-à-vis des apprenants
- L'accent a été mis sur l'apprentissage et non sur la stigmatisation des personnes qui ont fait des erreurs
- Les apprenants ont pu exprimer leurs réflexions et leurs ressentis sans crainte d'être mortifiés ou humiliés

Appendix 5: Agreement of the Ethics Committee of the Habib Thameur Hospital in Tunis to carry out the study

<table>
<tr>
<td>Tunisian Republic
Ministry of Health
Habib Thameur Hospital
Ethics Commitee</td>
<td>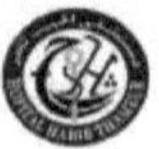</td>
<td dir="rtl">الجمهورية التونسية
وزارة الصحة
مستشفى الحبيب ثامر
لجنة الأخلاق</td>
</tr>
</table>

HABIB THAMEUR HOSPITAL
ETHICS COMMITTEE APPROVAL

Project title:

«Evaluation of learning of diagnostic digestive endoscopy by procedural simulation»

«Evaluation de l'apprentissage par la simulation procédurale en endoscopie digestive diagnostique»

Lead Principal Investigator: Dr Mariem SABBAH

Nature of Project: Prospective study

Local Chief Investigator: Pr Khadija MZOUGHI

Project Contact Point: phone: 00 216 98629843

Mail: sabbah_meriam@yahoo.fr

Supervisor: Pr Dalila GARGOURI

Hospital: Habib Thameur Hospital

Approval Number: *HTHEC-2019-34*

Members of Habib Thameur Hospital Ethics Committee (HTHEC).

Pr Dalila GARGOURI (MD, Chairperson), Pr Fatma BOUSSEMA (MD), Pr Sonia TRABELSI (MD), Pr Ag Ehsen Ben Brahim (MD), Pr Ag Zohra AYDI (MD), Dr Rabiaa BEN ABDALLAH (MD), Dr Asma BEN HASSEN (pharmacist), Dr Hela MAAMOURI (MD), Dr Aida Daib (MD), Mr Adel BEN HASSINE (lawyer), Mrs Ghofrane EZZINE (civil society, patient representative)

Date: 30/09/2019

Professor Dalila GARGOURI
Chairperson

Appendix 6: evaluation grid for simulation trainers (debriefing part) [27].

	Débriefing : phase descriptive			
17	Passer en revue les objectifs définis			
18	Préciser les étapes du débriefing et son déroulement			
19	Spécifier son rôle comme celui d'un facilitateur/animateur uniquement			
20	Communiquer sur ses attentes en termes d'auto-évaluation et d'évaluation de performance d'équipe			
21	Formuler des questions ouvertes			
22	Favoriser l'expression des étudiants			
23	Reconnaître les inquiétudes des apprenants au sujet du réalisme des situations simulées et les aider à apprendre, malgré les limites de la simulation			
24	Encourager les apprenants à exprimer leur ressenti et leurs émotions et à évacuer le stress provoqué par la simulation sans crainte d'être mortifiés ou humiliés			
25	Impliquer l'ensemble des apprenants			
26	Faire preuve de respect envers les apprenants			
27	Guider les échanges de façon à ce qu'ils progressent de façon logique plutôt que de passer d'un point à un autre sans cohérence			
28	Prendre compte des remarques des apprenants			

	Débriefing : phase d'analyse			
29	Fournir un feedback constructif aux apprenants à propos de leur performance individuelle ou collective en argumentant son point de vue			
30	Exposer ses propres raisonnements, sa perception de la situation			
31	Utiliser les actions observées comme base d'exploration et d'échanges			
32	Comparer la performance réalisée par les apprenants avec une performance attendue			
33	Explorer les raisons des différences entre performance réalisée et attendue			
34	Apporter les éléments théoriques nécessaires au réajustement des connaissances			
35	Poser des questions ouvertes			
36	Aider les apprenants à contextualiser leurs connaissances			
37	Utiliser des exemples concrets (pas seulement des commentaires abstraits ou généralistes) pour amener les apprenants à réfléchir sur leur performance			
38	Utiliser des propos clairs ; ne pas obliger les apprenants à imaginer ses pensées			
39	Ecouter et être attentif aux apprenants en reformulant leur propos, et en utilisant un langage non verbal adapté (par exemple, en regardant dans les yeux ou par des hochements de tête)			
40	Ne pas porter de jugement de valeur			
41	Ne pas tenir compte de propos discriminant			
42	Aider les apprenants à décontextualiser leurs connaissances pour pouvoir les généraliser, les appliquer et les transférer en pratique réelle			
43	Préciser les points forts de l'apprenant qu'il faut renforcer			
44	Préciser les points faibles à améliorer			
45	Identifier de nouveaux objectifs d'apprentissage pour les aider à combler les lacunes dans leurs connaissances			

46	Si l'un des apprenants s'est senti contrarié ou émotionnellement troublé lors du débriefing, être respectueux et constructif en l'aidant à gérer ses émotions			
47	Utiliser la vidéo ou d'autres enregistrements à bon escient comme support pour les échanges et l'apprentissage			
	Débriefing : phase de synthèse			
48	Passer en revue les points appris			
49	Aider les apprenants à faire des liens entre les différentes notions explorées			
50	Relier la séance de simulation aux façons dont les apprenants pourraient améliorer leur pratique clinique future			
51	Planifier la prochaine session ou la session de correction			
52	Donner un feedback aux apprenants sur la session dans son ensemble			
53	Remercier les apprenants pour leur participation			
54	Appréciation globale de la séance de simulation			
55	les objectifs pédagogiques sont atteints			
56	Le formateur a joué le rôle de facilitateur de l'apprentissage			
57	Le formateur a structuré le débriefing en 3 phases : réactions, analyse et synthèse			
58	Le formateur a adapté le niveau de facilitation au degré de participation des apprenants			
59	En cas de présence de 2 formateurs : coordination des tâches de chacun			

TABLE OF CONTENTS

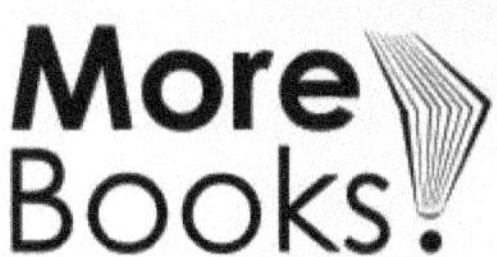

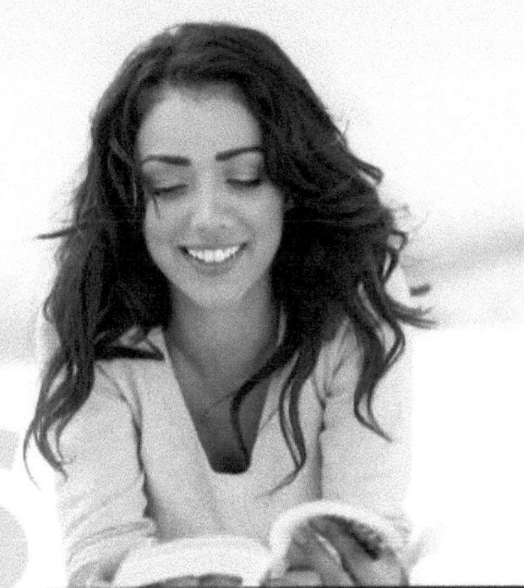

yes
I want morebooks!

Buy your books fast and straightforward online - at one of world's fastest growing online book stores! Environmentally sound due to Print-on-Demand technologies.

Buy your books online at
www.morebooks.shop

Kaufen Sie Ihre Bücher schnell und unkompliziert online – auf einer der am schnellsten wachsenden Buchhandelsplattformen weltweit! Dank Print-On-Demand umwelt- und ressourcenschonend produzi ert.

Bücher schneller online kaufen
www.morebooks.shop

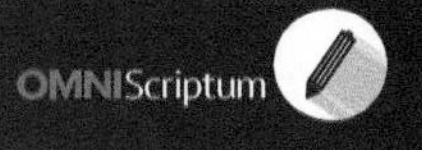

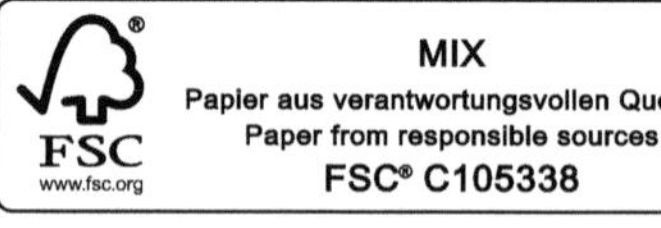

Printed by Books on Demand GmbH, Norderstedt / Germany